LIVING WITH ANXIETY

by Sheryl Normandeau

BrightPoint Press

San Diego, CA

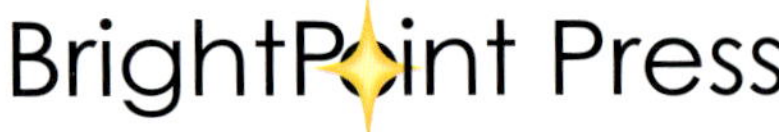

Content Consultant: Noam Shpancer, PhD, Professor of Psychology, Otterbein University

LIBRARY OF CONGRESS CATALOGING-IN-PUBLICATION DATA

Names: Normandeau, Sheryl, author.
Title: Living with anxiety / by Sheryl Normandeau.
Description: San Diego, CA: BrightPoint Press, [2024] | Series: Mental health support | Includes bibliographical references and index. | Audience: Ages 13 | Audience: Grades 7-9
Identifiers: LCCN 2023008670 (print) | LCCN 2023008671 (eBook) | ISBN 9781678206628 (hardcover) | ISBN 9781678206635 (eBook)
Subjects: LCSH: Anxiety in children--Juvenile literature. | Anxiety in adolescence--Juvenile literature. | Anxiety in children--Treatment--Juvenile literature. | Anxiety in adolescence--Treatment--Juvenile literature.
Classification: LCC RJ506.A58 .N67 2024 (print) | LCC RJ506.A58 (eBook) | DDC 618.92/8522--dc23/eng/20230417
LC record available at https://lccn.loc.gov/2023008670
LC eBook record available at https://lccn.loc.gov/2023008671

CONTENTS

AT A GLANCE

- People with anxiety disorders experience high levels of worry or fear. These feelings affect their daily lives.

- People with generalized anxiety disorder (GAD) experience symptoms of anxiety that last for long periods of time.

- Repeated panic attacks are the main symptom of panic disorder.

- Social anxiety disorder is a common type of anxiety disorder. People with this disorder fear being in situations where they may be judged negatively by others.

- People with specific phobias experience intense anxiety about certain objects or situations.

- Some people experience anxiety when they are separated from their loved ones. They may be diagnosed with separation anxiety.

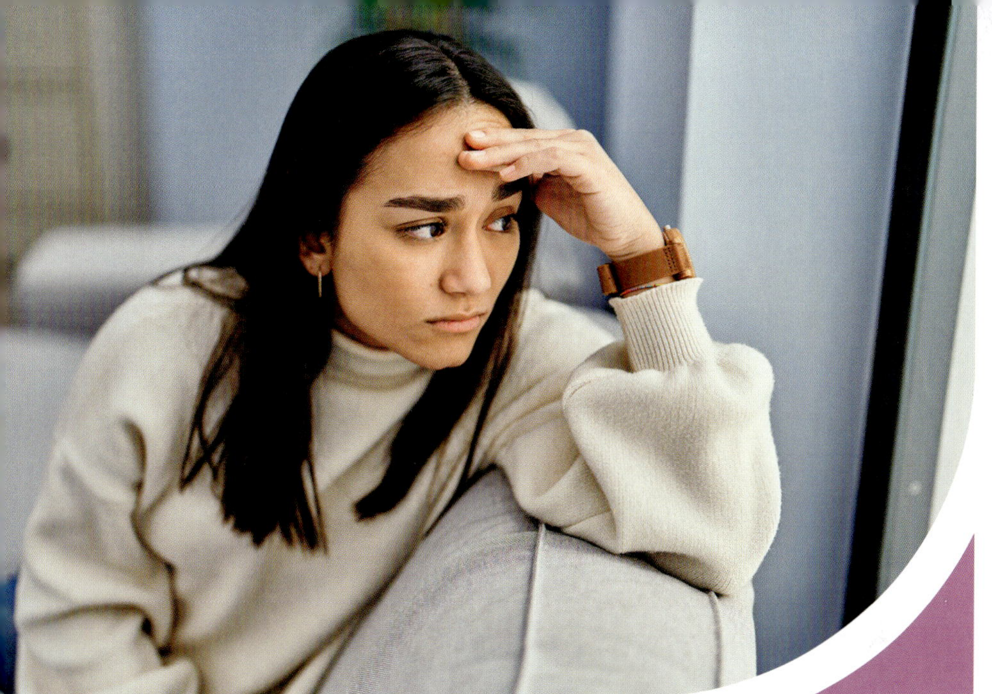

- Therapy such as cognitive behavioral therapy (CBT), which includes exposure therapy, is often used to treat anxiety disorders. Dialectical behavior therapy (DBT) and acceptance and commitment therapy can also be used.

- Medication is one way to treat anxiety disorders. Antidepressants, benzodiazepines, and beta-blockers can help manage anxiety.

- Lifestyle changes, such as exercise and a healthy diet, can be helpful for people with anxiety disorders. These changes can boost the effects of medication or therapy.

INTRODUCTION

A NEW SCHOOL

Naya just started sixth grade in a new school. The move is a huge change. She feels like she does not fit in. She is having a hard time making friends. She misses her friends from her old school. Naya used to be a good student. But now she is having trouble concentrating. Her grades have fallen.

Naya has a hard time sleeping. She worries about going to school. Sometimes

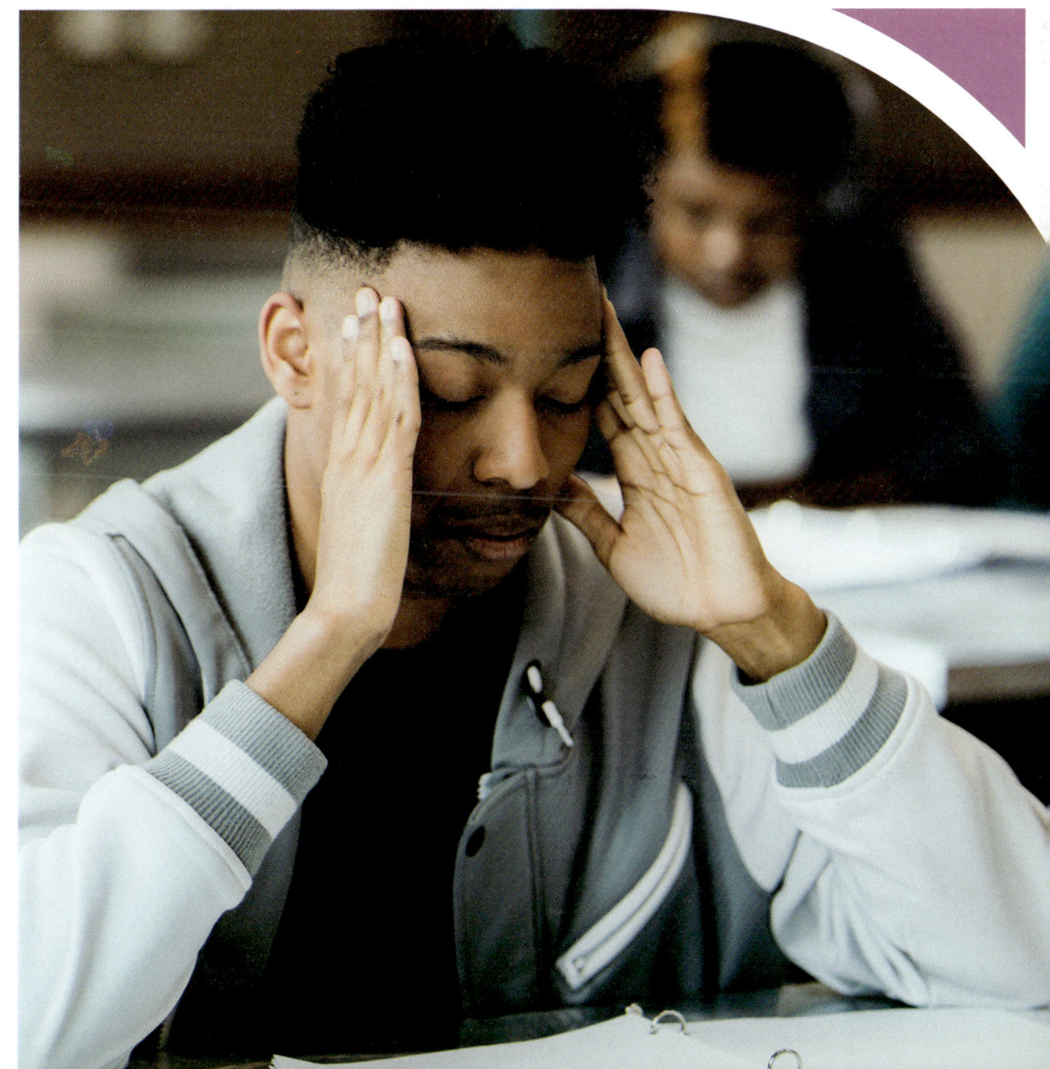

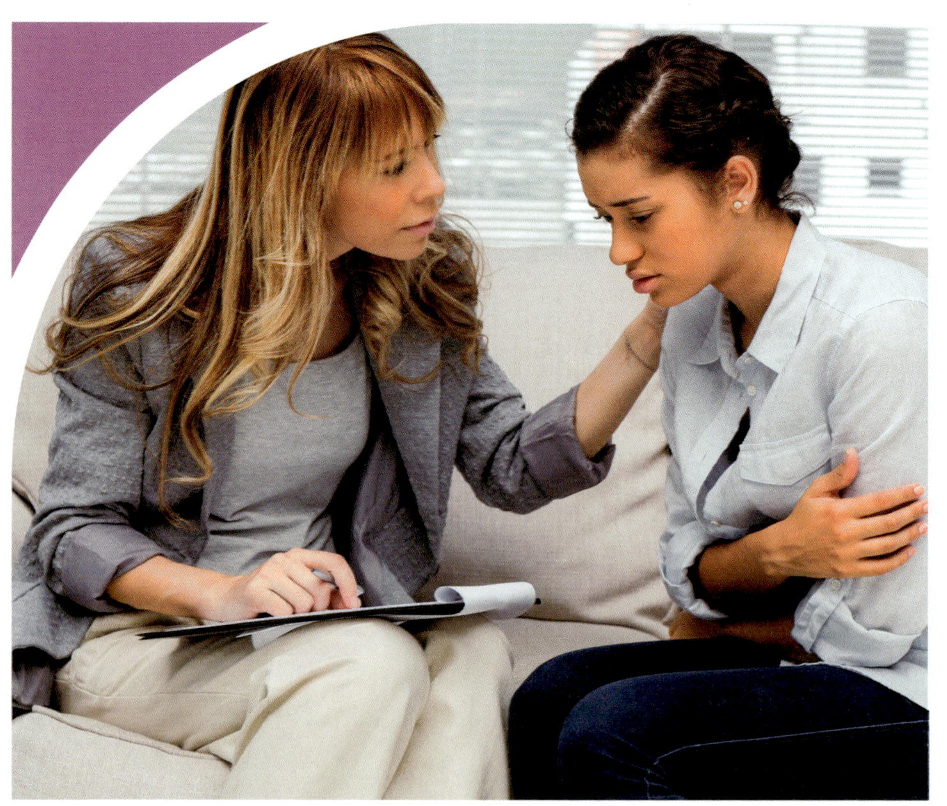

School guidance counselors can help students cope with anxiety.

her stomach hurts so badly she feels like

throwing up.

Naya's parents noticed her change in

behavior. They asked her about her feelings.

Naya's teachers saw she was struggling

with schoolwork. They suggested she speak to the school's guidance counselor. Naya learned she was dealing with anxiety.

Naya's family, teachers, and school counselor supported her. She began to see a therapist. He helped Naya with her anxiety. Naya also tried deep-breathing exercises. Over time, she started feeling better.

WHAT IS ANXIETY?

Anxiety is a feeling of worry or fear. Most people experience these emotions from time to time. And a certain level of anxiety

can help people stay alert and safe. But
these feelings are overwhelming for people
with anxiety disorders. Anxiety makes it
difficult for them to go to school or try new
things. People may spend less time with
their friends and families.

Dr. Anne Marie Albano is the director
of the Clinic for Anxiety and Related
Disorders. She described how anxiety
differs from nervousness. "It should feel
like butterflies in your stomach when you're
asking someone you like out for a date.
And it should feel like your heart pounding if
you're being called on in front of the whole

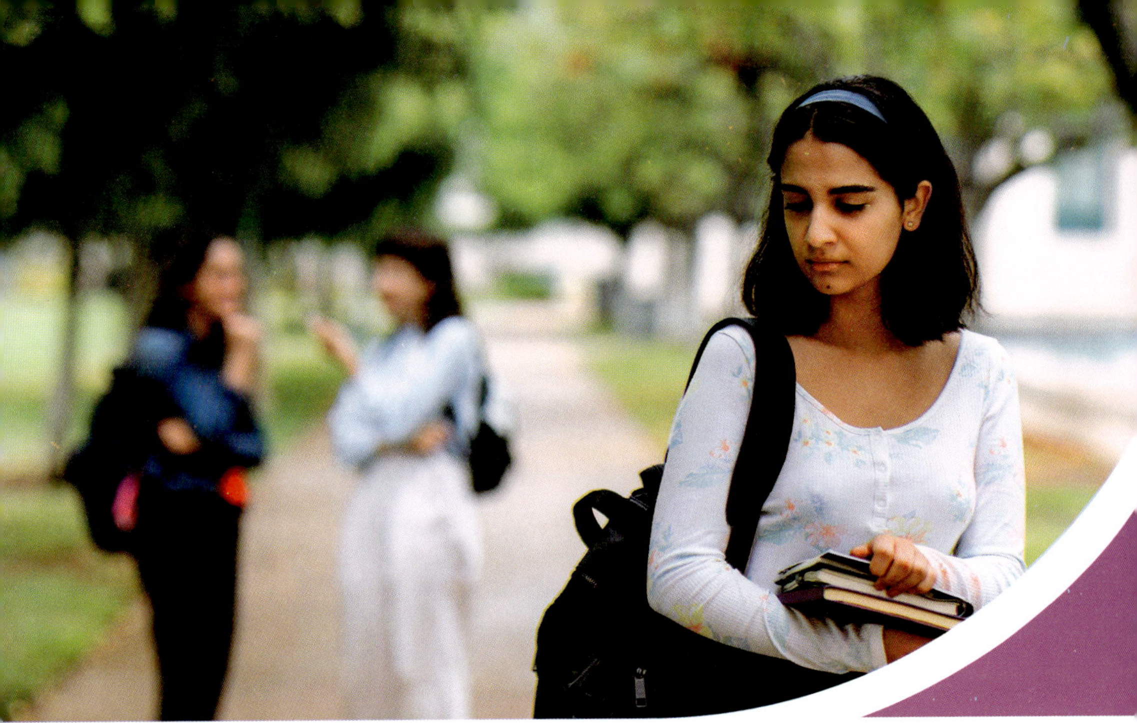

Some people with anxiety may struggle to make new friends.

class," she said. "But it shouldn't overwhelm you . . . so much that you can't turn it off."[1]

Fortunately, there are ways to treat anxiety disorders. Therapy, medication, and lifestyle changes can reduce anxiety. These treatments help people manage their **symptoms**.

1

HOW DOES ANXIETY FEEL?

Anxiety has many symptoms. They include feeling tense, restless, and tired. Difficulty concentrating and changes in sleep are other symptoms. People with anxiety may feel easily frustrated. Anxiety can also have physical effects. People may have a headache or a stomachache.

People may experience some or all of these symptoms.

Anxiety affects daily life. It can cause changes in behavior. People may spend less time with family and friends. They may struggle at school or at work.

People may experience a racing heartbeat when they feel anxious.

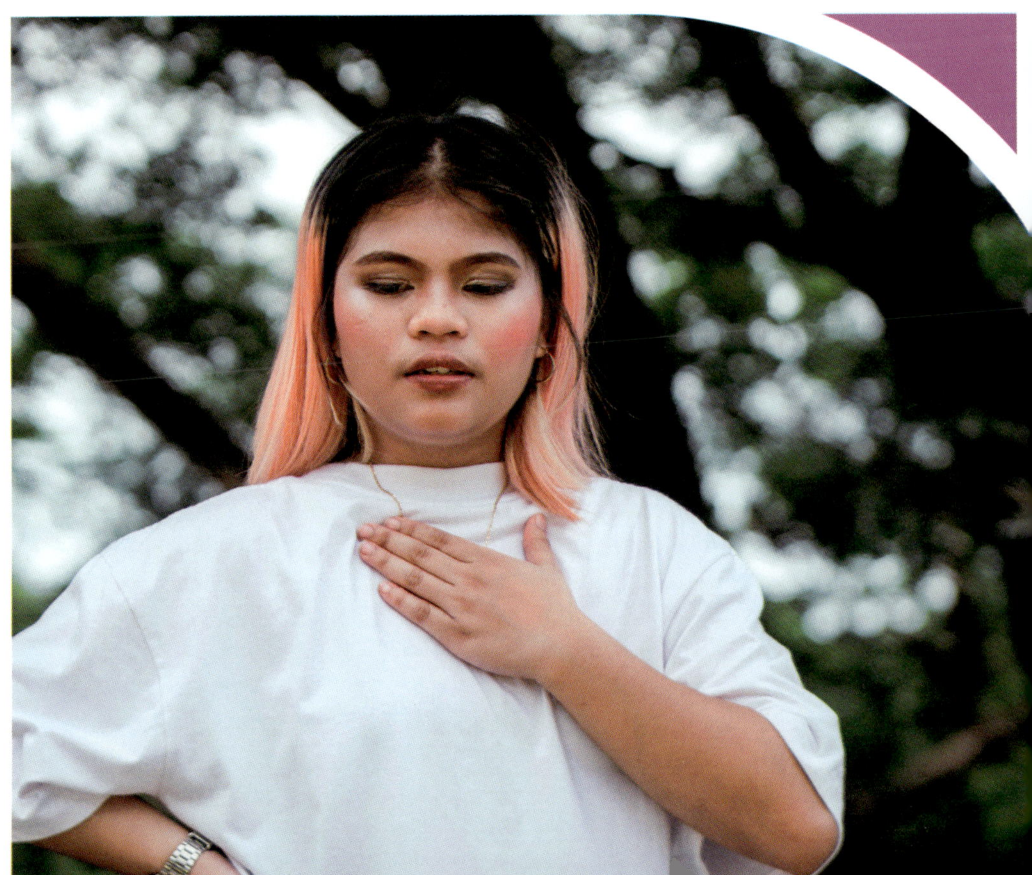

THE BODY'S RESPONSE TO DANGER

The amygdala is part of the human brain. It processes emotions, including fear. It alerts the body to danger. It starts the fight-or-flight response. This prepares the body to fight or run from threats.

High stress levels can start the fight-or-flight response. The body releases a **hormone** called adrenaline. It is released from the adrenal glands. These glands are located above the kidneys. Adrenaline causes the heart to beat faster. It increases blood flow to the muscles. This prepares them to respond quickly.

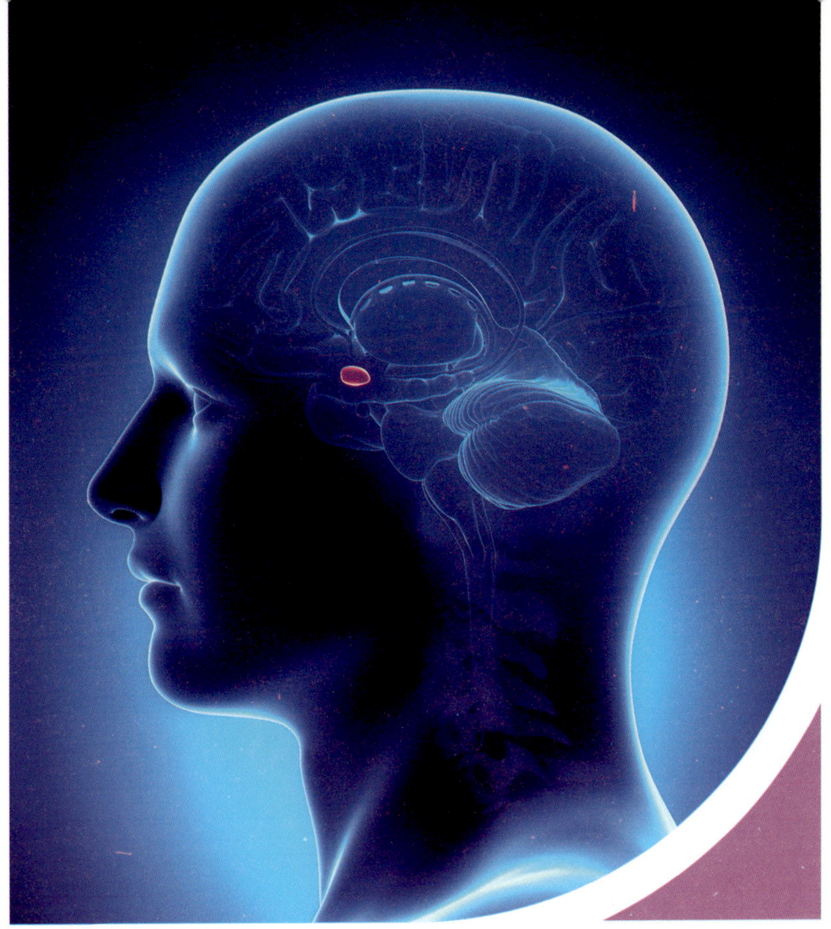

Sometimes this response remains active for a long time. People may experience anxiety. The amygdala may be overactive in people with an anxiety disorder. They may have high levels of adrenaline.

RISK FACTORS

Risk factors make it more likely for someone to develop an anxiety disorder. These disorders often run in families. A parent may have an anxiety disorder. The child then has a higher risk of developing an anxiety disorder too.

The environment someone was raised in is another factor. Abuse increases the risk. Other stressful events are also risk factors. These events include the death of a loved one. Moving to a new city or changing schools can cause anxiety.

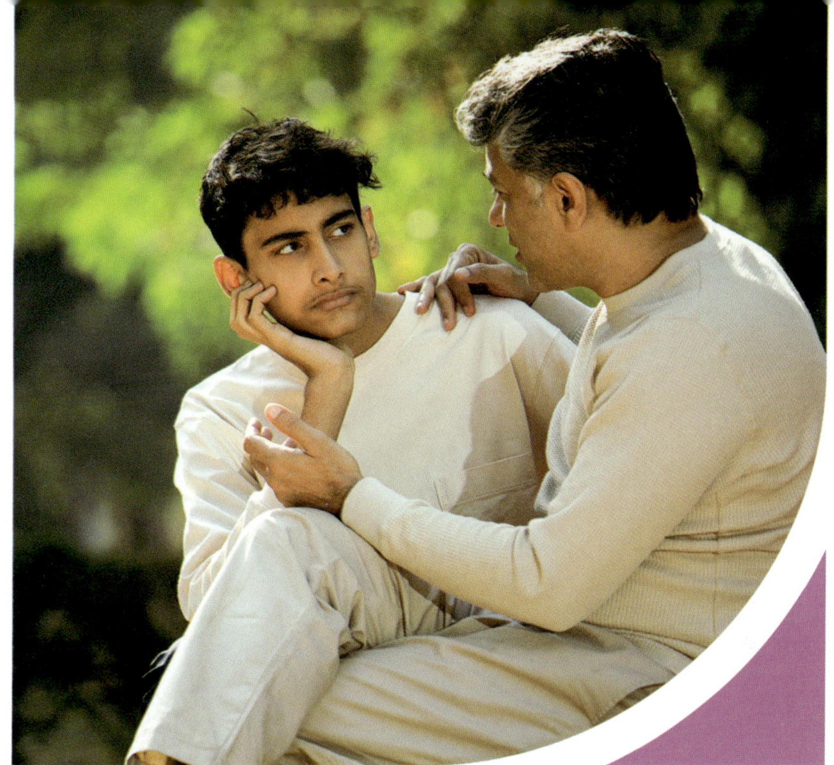

Natural disasters and wars can lead to the development of anxiety disorders.

Some medications have side effects. These side effects may be similar to symptoms of anxiety. Doctors rule out the

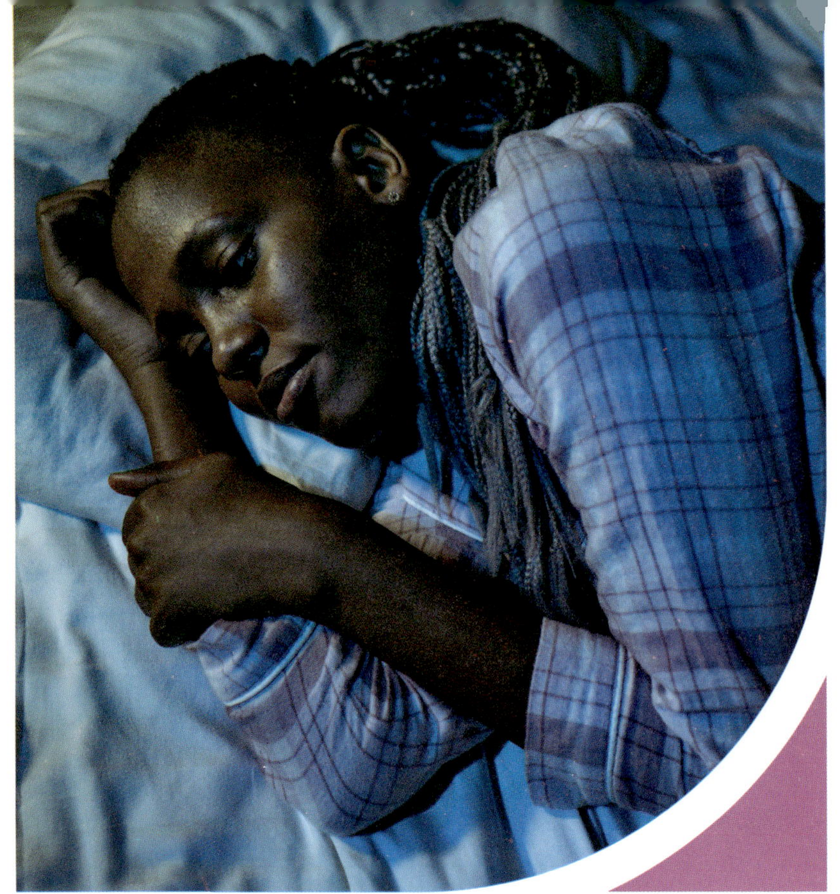

Anxiety can make it difficult to fall asleep.

effects of medications before making an anxiety disorder **diagnosis**.

TYPES OF ANXIETY

Anxiety disorders are the most common mental health disorders in the United States.

They affect more than 19 percent of the
population. Approximately 5.8 million
US children between the ages of three and
seventeen were diagnosed with an anxiety
disorder between 2016 and 2019.

There are several types of anxiety
disorders. People with generalized anxiety
disorder (GAD) experience high levels of
worry for months or years. The stress
affects their daily lives.

Other people may have panic disorder.
People with this disorder have repeated
panic attacks. They may feel scared,
weak, or nauseous during a panic attack.

They may have a rapid heartbeat and difficulty breathing. J. T. Lewis described the first time she had a panic attack. "Suddenly, I couldn't breathe," Lewis remembered. "There was this crushing chest pain. I knew something was terribly wrong. Was I dying?"[2]

Social anxiety disorder is a common anxiety disorder. It affects approximately 7 percent of the US population. This disorder often develops in teenagers. People with social anxiety fear being judged negatively by others. They may struggle with public speaking. They may avoid parties.

HOW COMMON ARE ANXIETY DISORDERS?

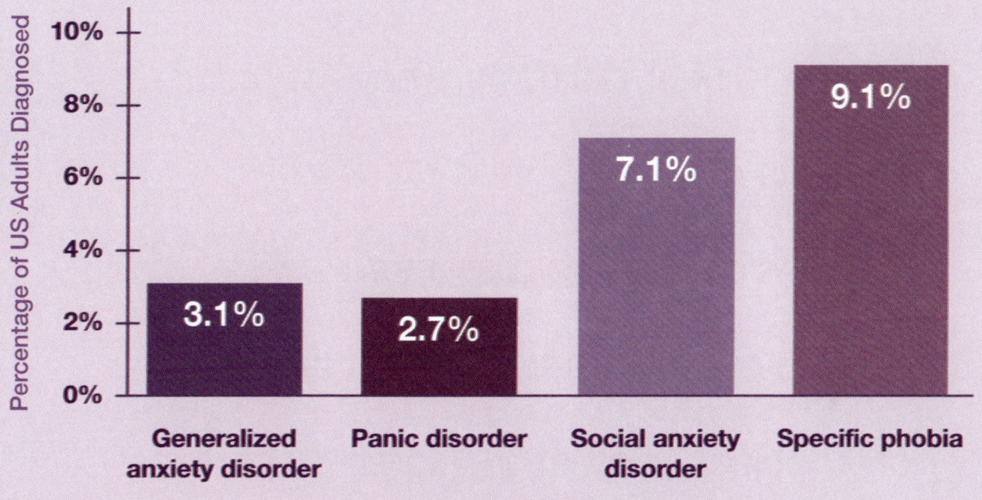

Source: "Anxiety Disorders Facts and Statistics," ADAA, October 28, 2022. https://adaa.org.

This graph shows the approximate percentage of US adults who are diagnosed with anxiety disorders. People may be diagnosed with multiple disorders.

They may feel anxious when eating in front of others. Social anxiety can make it difficult to go to school or work. Symptoms of this disorder include a rapid heartbeat and sweating. Social anxiety in children may include temper tantrums. They may refuse to talk to others.

Some people are diagnosed with a specific phobia. A phobia is an extreme fear of an object or situation. Common phobias include a fear of spiders. A fear of heights is also common. People with specific phobias have extreme anxiety when they come across the feared object or situation. They will go to great lengths to avoid their fears. This can affect daily life and health. For example, someone may have a phobia of needles. She may avoid going to the doctor because she does not want to get

a shot.

Separation anxiety is another type

of anxiety disorder. People fear being

separated from their loved ones. They

worry that something bad will happen to

those they care about. This disorder is most

AGORAPHOBIA

More than 1 percent of US adults experience agoraphobia. People with agoraphobia fear being in places where escape may be difficult. Crowds and public transport can cause anxiety. People may worry that they will not receive help if they have a panic attack. People with severe agoraphobia may be unable to leave home because of their anxiety. They may worry about having a panic attack in public.

common in young children. But teens and
adults can also be diagnosed with it.

HOW IS ANXIETY DIAGNOSED?

Talking about anxiety can be difficult.
But asking for help is the first step to
recovery. Many states have mental health
hotlines. People can call to speak to trained
professionals. They can receive resources
such as contact information for doctors
or therapists.

Parents and teachers may notice that a
child is having symptoms of anxiety. These
adults can help find a doctor or mental

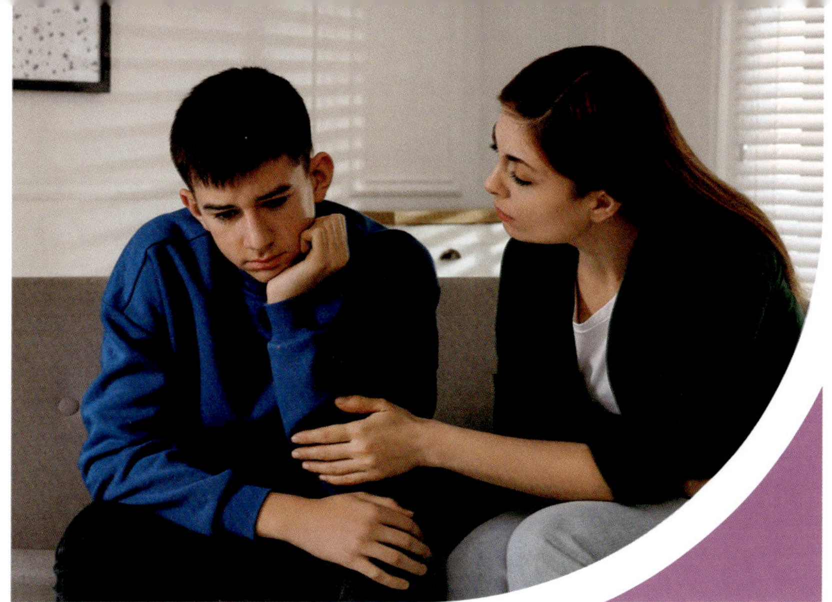

health professional. A child may go see

a therapist or psychiatrist. These medical

professionals assess the child's symptoms.

They determine whether the symptoms are

caused by an anxiety disorder. Therapists

and psychiatrists also treat anxiety

disorders. Psychiatrists can **prescribe**

medication to help with anxiety.

2
THERAPIES TO TREAT ANXIETY

Many people with anxiety disorders find relief through therapy. Therapy can be paired with medication. Or people may choose therapy alone to manage anxiety.

Patients describe their symptoms to a mental health professional during therapy. They work together to find ways to manage anxiety. Patients learn to cope with their symptoms in a healthy way.

Therapy can be done in several ways. A patient may speak to a mental health professional in a one-on-one session. Or a

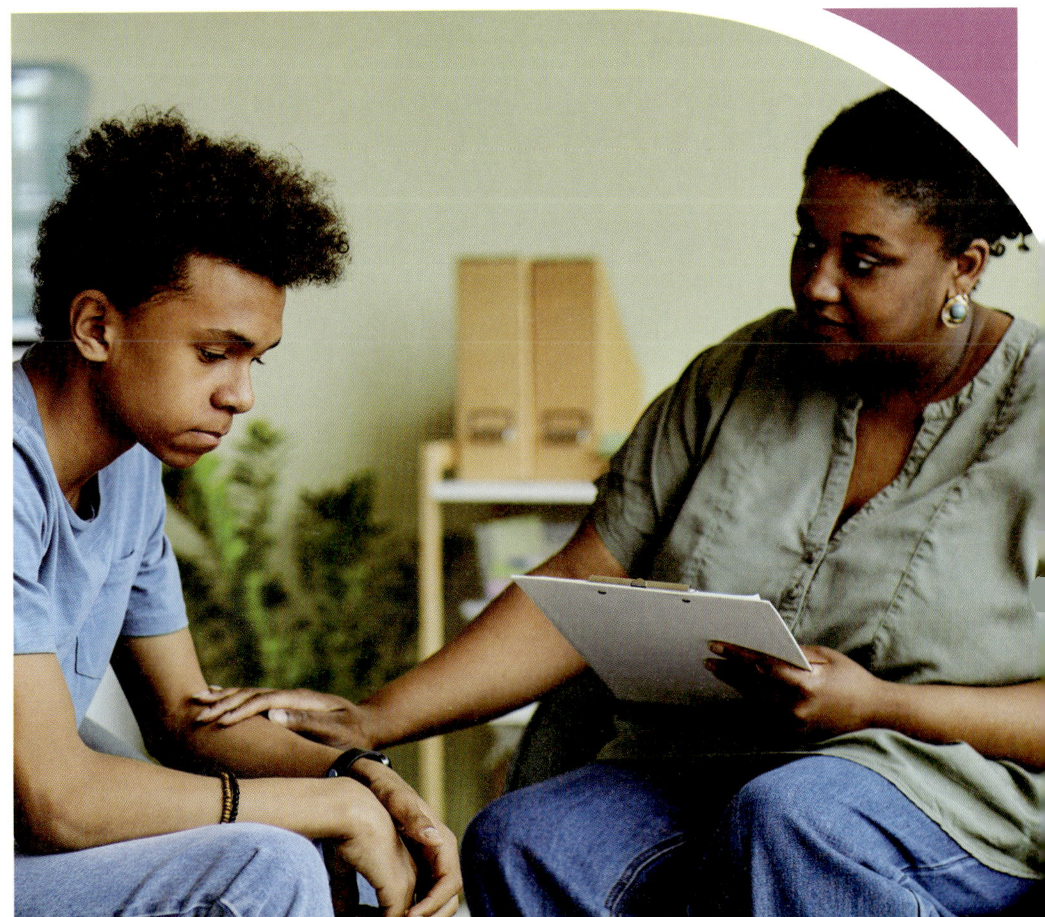

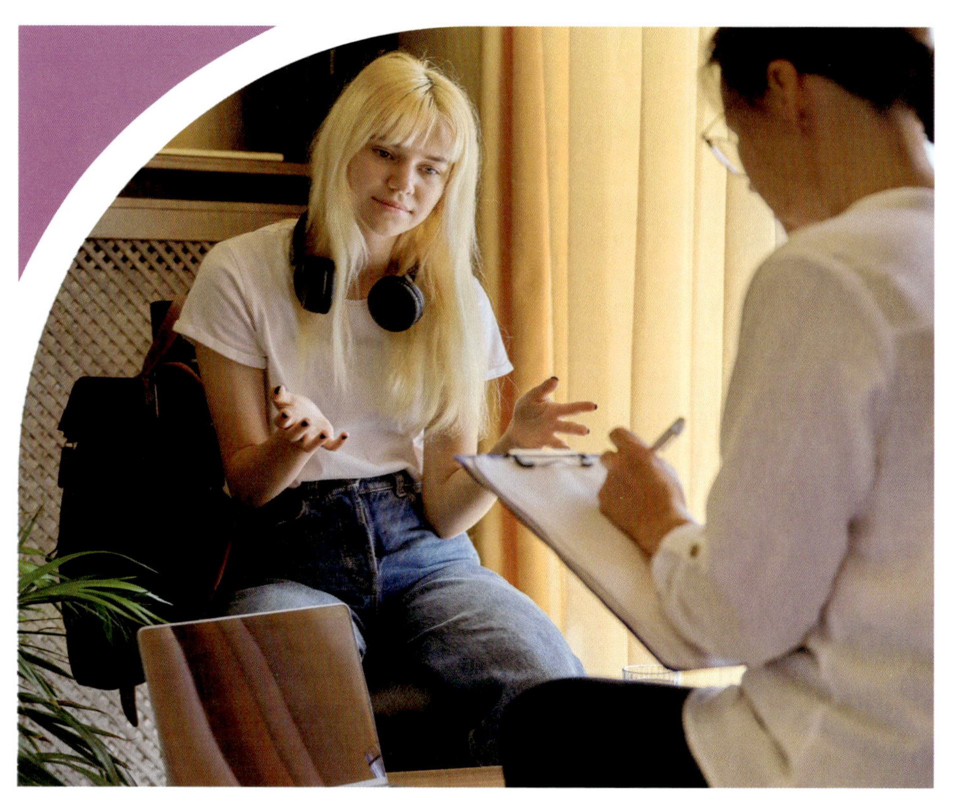

People should feel comfortable discussing sensitive subjects with their therapist.

group of patients with similar struggles may

meet together with a trained professional.

Family members may also see a therapist

together. Therapy can be administered

online or in person.

There are many types of therapies that can treat anxiety. Some are effective for all types of anxiety disorders. Others work best for certain anxiety disorders.

COGNITIVE BEHAVIORAL THERAPY

Cognitive behavioral therapy (CBT) is the most common therapy used to treat anxiety disorders. People with anxiety may have negative thought patterns. These thoughts can feel overwhelming and add to their stress. For example, someone may have had a negative experience at the dentist. This may have caused him to develop a phobia of dentists. He may think that all visits to the dentist will be painful.

CBT helps people adjust their thinking. Therapists teach patients to recognize unhelpful and inaccurate thoughts. Patients learn to replace negative thought patterns with positive and accurate thinking. The person with the dentist phobia may work to remember past trips that were not painful.

Matt Grammer is a counselor. Grammer described how CBT works. He said, "[CBT] helps because negative thoughts cause . . . negative emotions, which lead to destructive behaviors. CBT focuses on

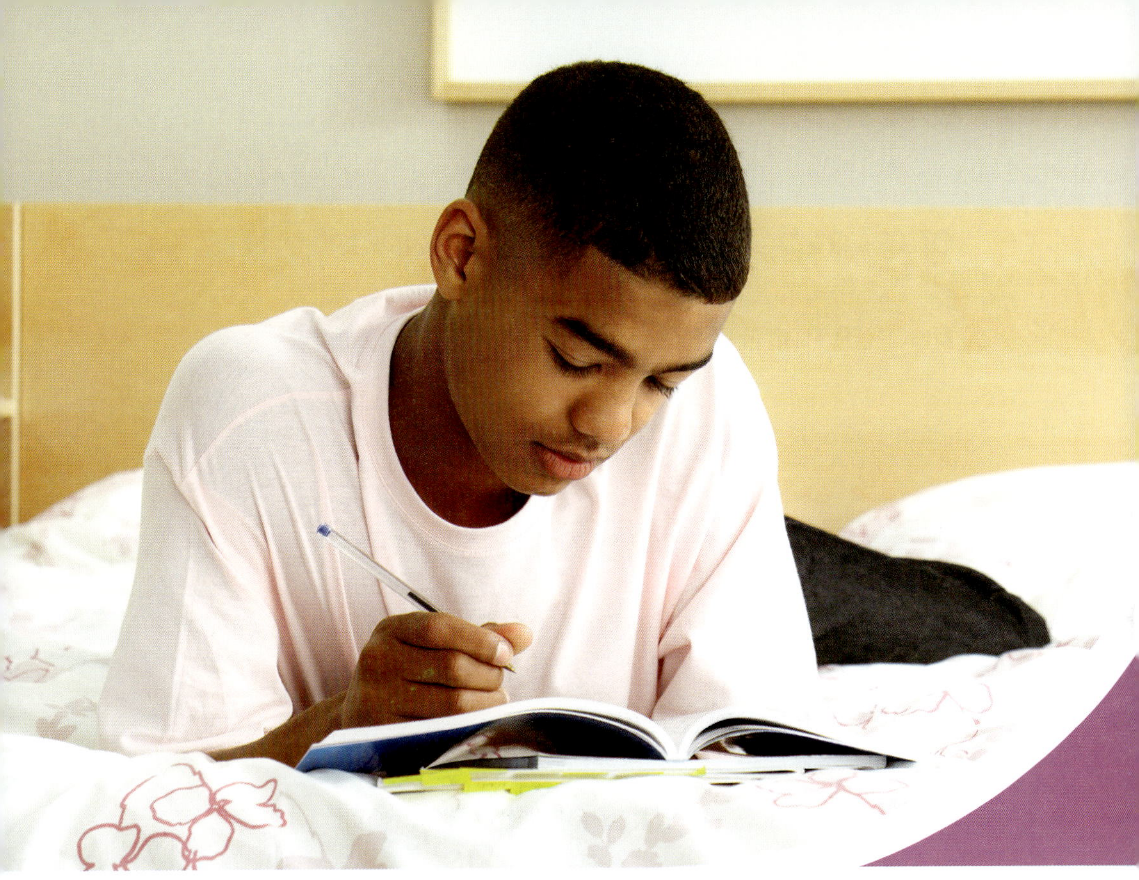

identifying unhealthy thought processes

and . . . [stopping] them from escalating to

feelings of anxiety."[3]

CBT also focuses on patients'

behaviors. People with anxiety disorders

often avoid tasks that cause anxiety. This negatively affects their lives. Therapists help their clients face their fears. They teach patients to manage emotions. This may involve deep-breathing and muscle relaxation exercises.

Dialectical behavior therapy (DBT) has similarities to CBT. DBT helps people understand and accept their symptoms. It trains people to recognize ways they can improve their mental health. DBT teaches skills that help people manage anxiety and emotions. For example, patients may work on setting boundaries or asking for help.

EXPOSURE THERAPY

Exposure therapy is often used to treat specific phobias. But this therapy can help with other anxiety disorders too. It is often a part of CBT. People are gradually exposed to the object or situation that gives them

ACCEPTANCE AND COMMITMENT THERAPY

Acceptance and commitment therapy is a new form of therapy. Therapists help patients think about their values. Patients accept and pay attention to their thoughts. They practice mindfulness. Patients learn to understand their values and motivations. This can encourage positive behavior.

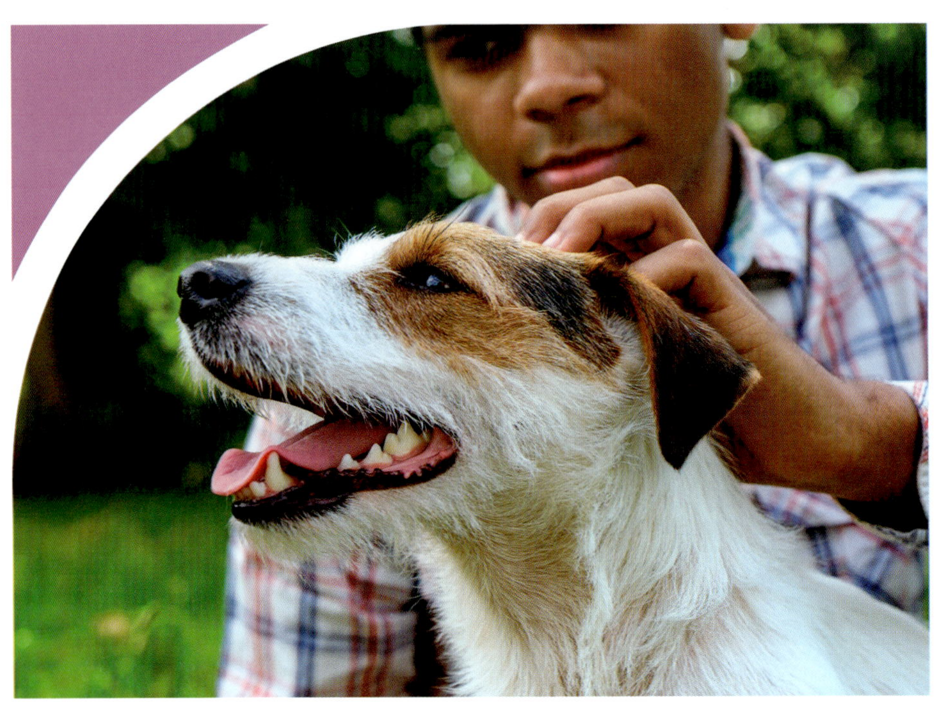

Someone who has a phobia of dogs may work with a therapist so that he can pet a dog without feeling severe anxiety.

anxiety. Therapists work with patients. They work to develop skills to manage anxiety.

People receiving exposure therapy create a list of goals. The goals are related to their anxiety. They rank the goals from least to most challenging. Therapists and patients work to accomplish the easy goals first.

For example, someone may have a fear of

spiders. Her first goal may be to learn to

manage anxiety when she thinks about a

spider. Then she might look at a picture of

a spider. Eventually she may want to be in

the same room as a spider without feeling

overwhelming fear.

Sometimes therapists use a flooding

technique during exposure therapy.

Therapists make sure patients have the

tools to manage their anxiety. Then they

expose patients to the feared object in a

controlled environment. This technique can

help someone overcome a phobia quickly.

But it can be scary at first.

GROUP THERAPY

Some people benefit from group therapy.

Group therapy can remind people that they

are not alone. Other people have similar

experiences with anxiety. People in the

group support one another. Members may

share ways they manage their anxiety.

Group therapy can be especially effective

for people with social anxiety disorder.

Kevin Chapman is a clinical psychologist.

He talked about how group therapy helps

treat social anxiety. "[Group therapy]

actually works as a part of exposure

therapy because a support group is in its

nature a social setting," he said. "It's an

extremely safe place to open up about your

experience because you know the others

there are experiencing it too."[4]

SERVICE DOGS

Pets can reduce anxiety. Service dogs are trained to help people with anxiety and other mental health disorders. They can be trained to notice signs of a panic attack. They can bring medication to owners. Service dogs can also help calm a person down. They may lick the owner's face to try to get his or her attention. This may alert them that something is wrong.

3
TREATING ANXIETY WITH MEDICATION

A doctor or psychiatrist may prescribe medication to treat an anxiety disorder. There are different types of medications for anxiety. These include antidepressants, benzodiazepines, and beta-blockers. The medicine and **dose** vary from person to person. Doctors and patients work together to find a medication that

manages symptoms.

Medication does not work for everybody. Some people do not respond well to it. Medication can also cause side effects.

Doctors and patients should discuss side effects of medication before starting use.

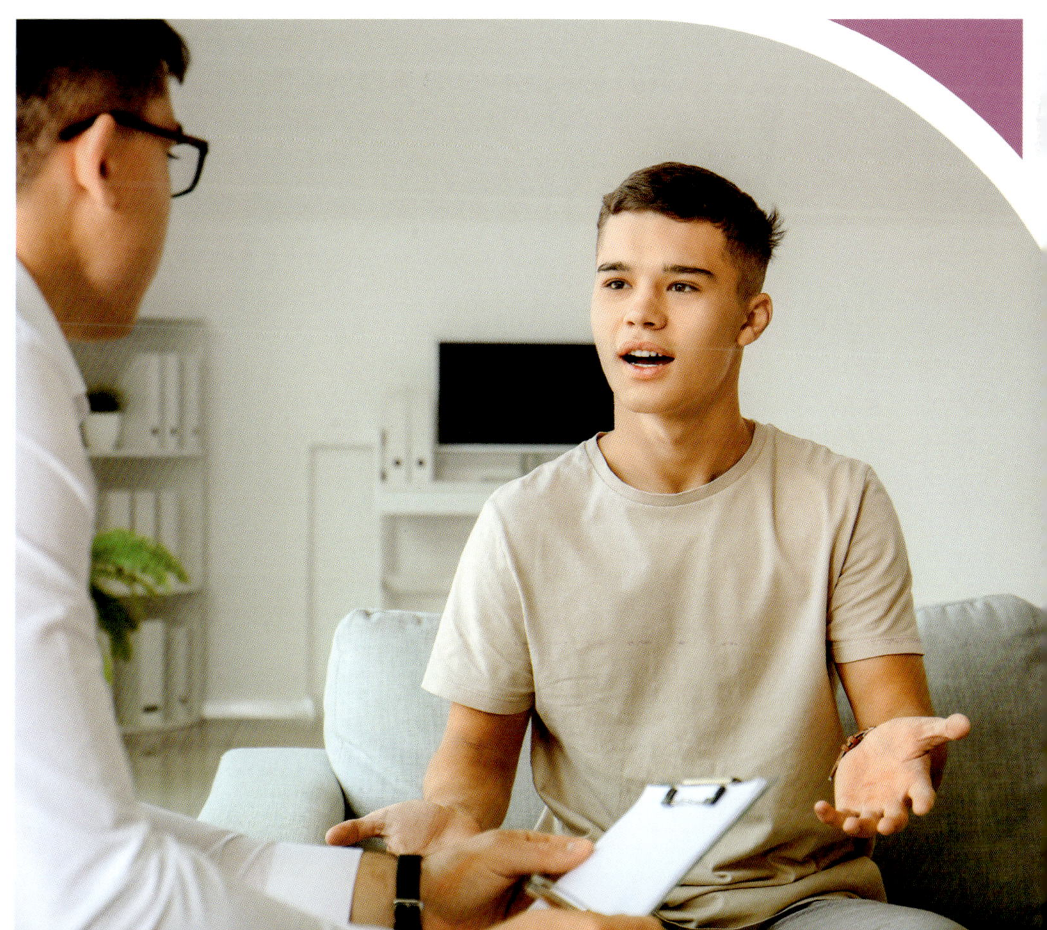

Side effects vary depending on the drug. They include dry mouth, drowsiness, and nausea. Patients should speak to their doctors about side effects. They also need to talk to their doctors if they want to stop treatment. It is not safe to suddenly stop taking certain anxiety medications. Doctors will work with patients on how to safely stop use.

ANTIDEPRESSANTS

Antidepressants are often used to treat depression. They can also be used to treat anxiety disorders. Selective serotonin

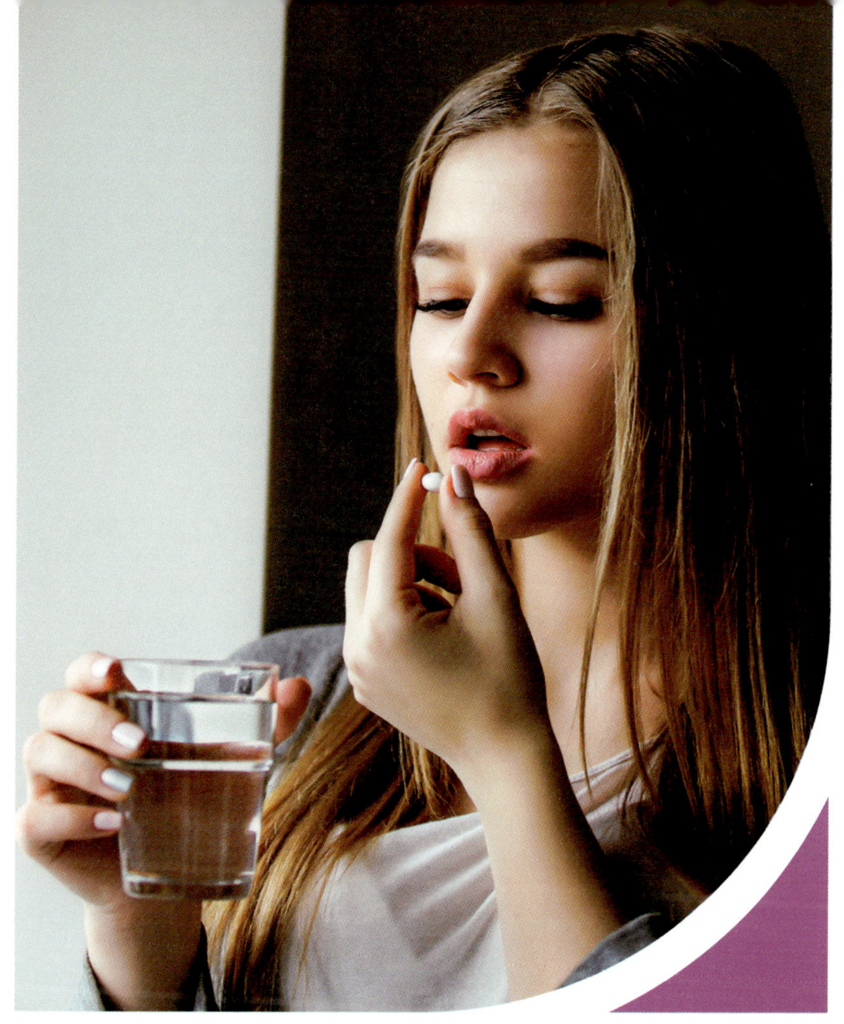

reuptake inhibitors (SSRIs) are a type of

antidepressant that can treat anxiety.

Serotonin is a **neurotransmitter**. It

affects mood.

Selective norepinephrine reuptake inhibitors (SNRIs) are another antidepressant. They increase levels of norepinephrine in the brain. Many people have found relief from anxiety symptoms after taking SNRIs.

Doctors often prescribe SSRIs and SNRIs to treat anxiety. These drugs are not **addictive**. They are also effective in treating all types of anxiety disorders. But these drugs can take several weeks to work. Dr. Evelyn Stewart studies mental health. She spoke of the need for patience when taking anxiety medication. She said, "With

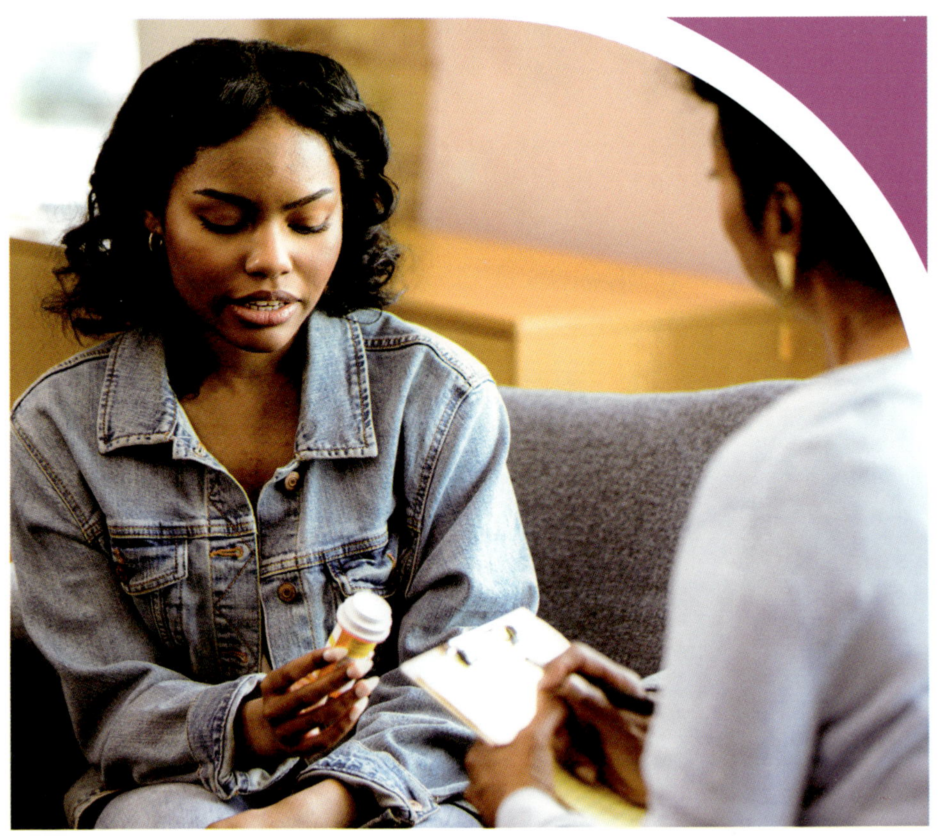

Patients should talk to their doctors if they want to stop using an anxiety medication.

treating anxiety . . . the treatment tends to be at least six months to a year. . . . But very often, even after that amount of time, youth who are feeling so much better are hesitant to stop the medication."[5]

BENZODIAZEPINES

Benzodiazepines are another type of anxiety medication. These drugs work much faster than SSRIs and SNRIs. People may feel the effects of the medicine in less than two hours. These drugs are usually prescribed to treat short-term anxiety issues. For example, people may have a

BUSPIRONE

Buspirone is used to treat GAD. It affects the levels of serotonin. The drug takes about a month to take effect. Buspirone is not addictive. But people may still experience mild side effects. They may feel dizzy or have a headache. Buspirone may be less effective if a person has taken benzodiazepines before.

fear of flying. They may experience high levels of anxiety before a flight. They can take a benzodiazepine before traveling.

Benzodiazepines treat many anxiety disorders, including panic disorder. But doctors do not often prescribe this medication. It can cause side effects such as drowsiness. People may have memory problems. Benzodiazepines become less effective over time. They are also addictive. People may experience **withdrawal** symptoms when they stop use. They may begin to feel tired and dizzy. It is important to take benzodiazepines as prescribed.

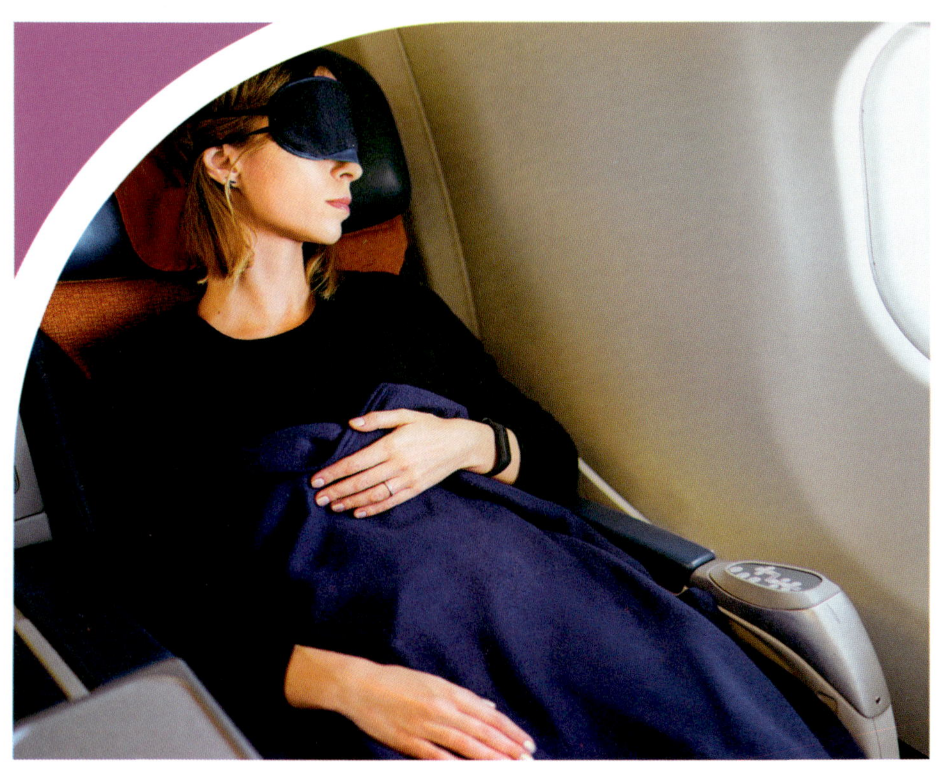

Doctors recommend that these drugs be

taken for fewer than two weeks.

BETA-BLOCKERS

Beta-blockers are typically prescribed to

treat heart conditions. But they can also

treat social anxiety disorder. Beta-blockers limit the effect of adrenaline on the heart. They prevent the heart from beating rapidly. They can reduce other physical symptoms of anxiety, such as sweating and dizziness.

Like benzodiazepines, beta-blockers take effect within a couple of hours. But beta-blockers tend to have fewer side effects. They are also less addictive. However, beta-blockers may not be effective against severe anxiety.

4
LIFESTYLE CHANGES TO REDUCE ANXIETY

Exercise, sleep, and a healthy diet can reduce anxiety. Meditation can also be helpful. Lifestyle changes can boost the effects of medication and therapy.

Ken Duckworth teaches psychiatry at Harvard Medical School in Boston, Massachusetts. He talked about the importance of lifestyle changes. He

said, "Some people will get better with

[therapy] alone. . . . Some people might

need medication to help them concentrate

[on therapy]. Anxiety . . . can decrease

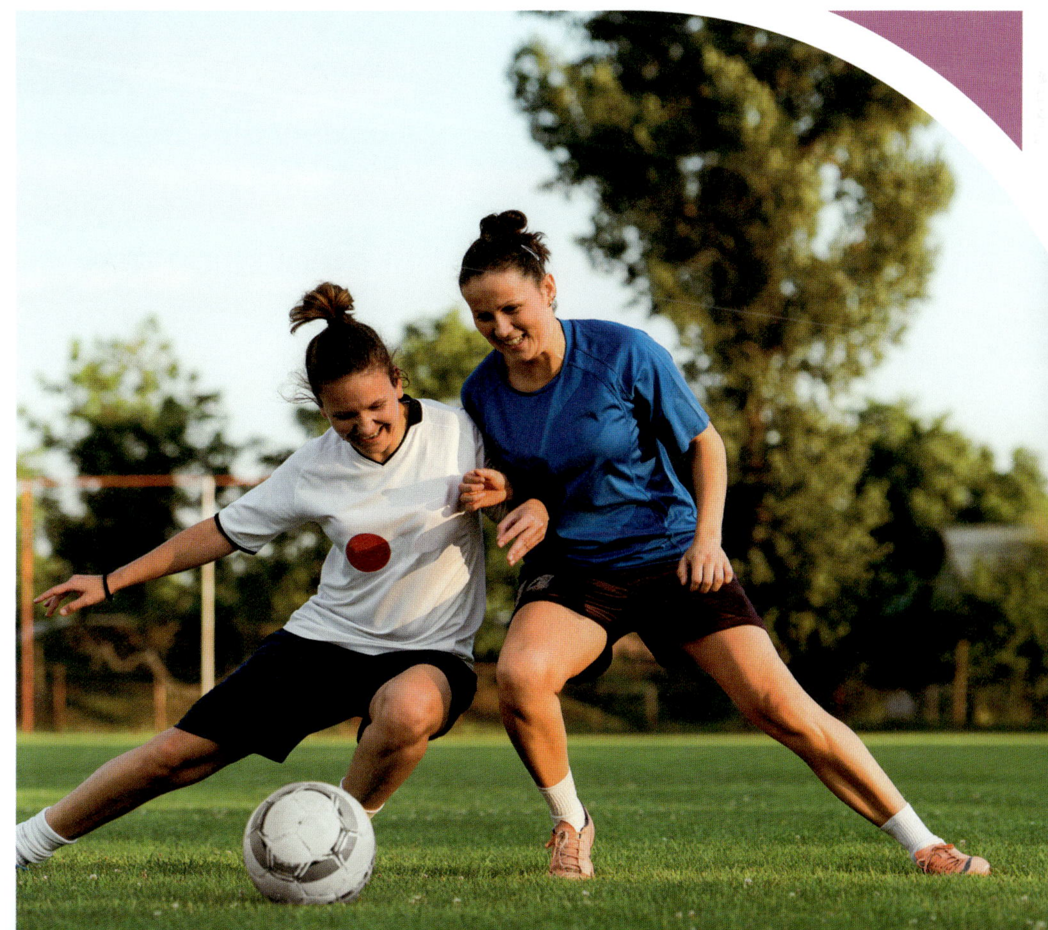

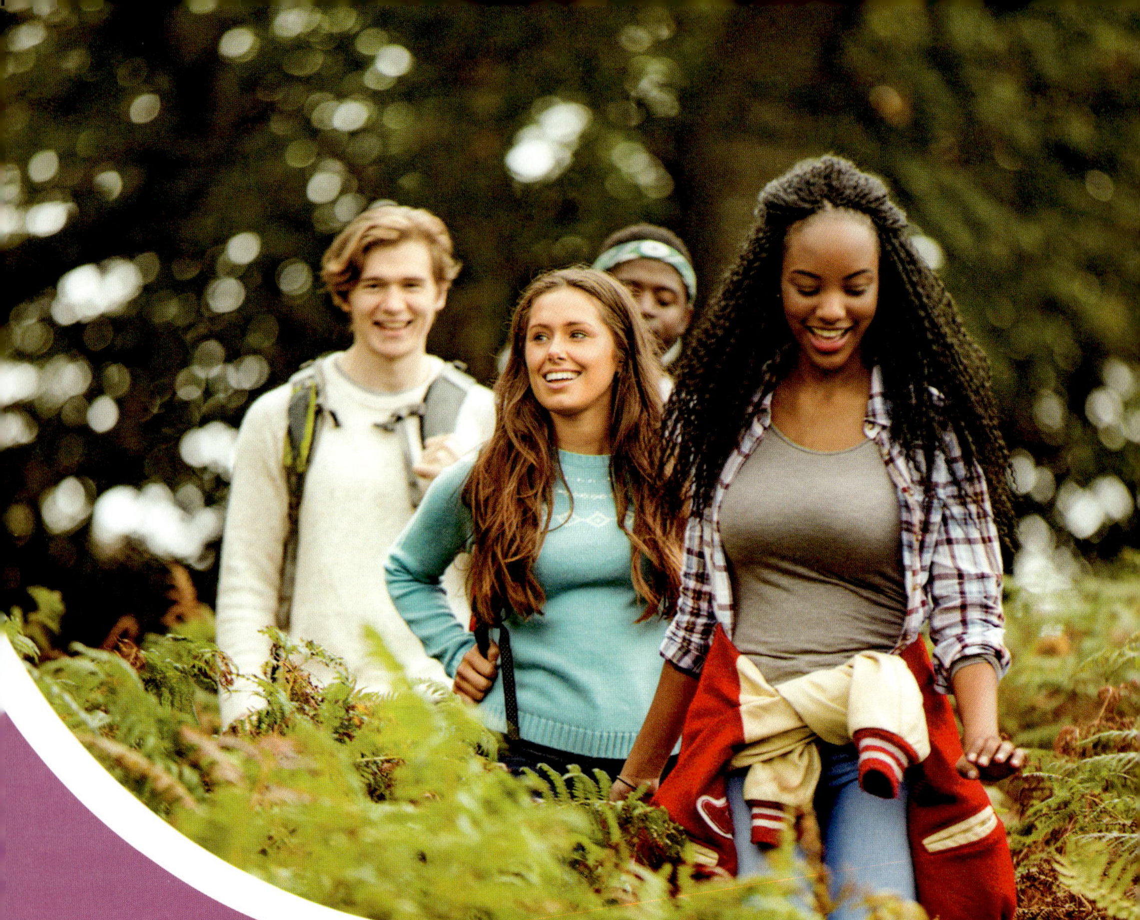

motivation to exercise, but medication may give you the energy to do it."[6]

Many doctors recommend regular exercise to reduce anxiety. Muscles become tense when people are stressed.

Exercise loosens muscles. It can also influence activity in the amygdala. This can reduce stress. Physical activity also increases heart rate. People with anxiety can learn to connect this feeling with exercise instead of anxiety.

Exercise encourages people to spend time outdoors. Studies show that being in nature reduces anxiety. It can lower stress levels. Spending time outdoors has other mental health benefits too. It can improve attention and concentration.

Exercise brings people into contact with others. They may play on a team or train

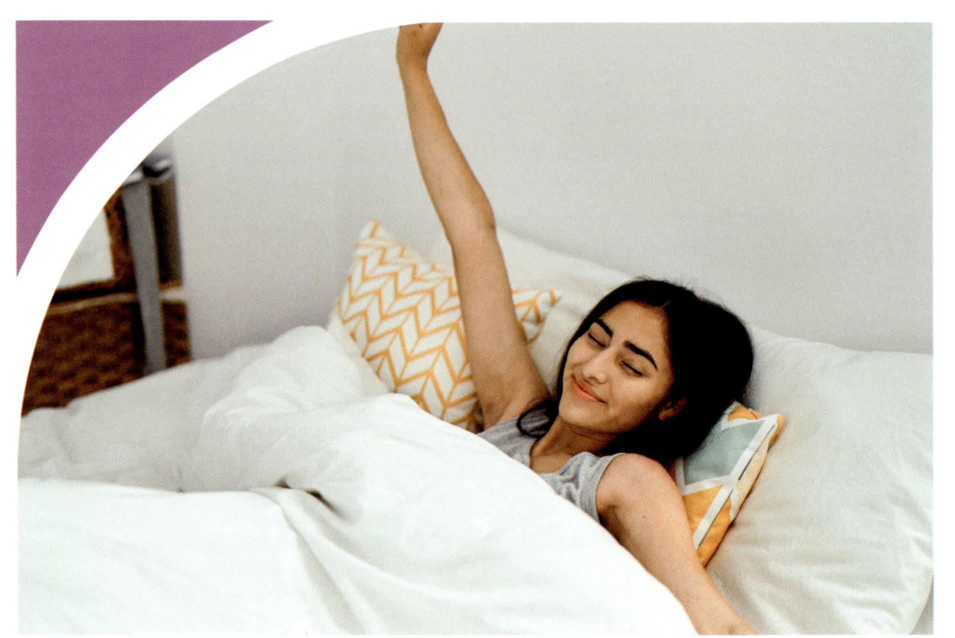

with friends. Social connections help people

cope with anxiety.

SLEEP

Getting enough sleep improves mental

health. Experts recommend getting an

average of eight hours of sleep every night.

Stress hormones may rise when people do not sleep enough. This can make anxiety worse. Sleep can improve memory and concentration. It helps the body fight off illness.

People can make changes to their nightly routines to help them sleep better. Having a set bedtime helps. People can avoid looking at screens before bedtime. A dark and quiet bedroom also helps.

HEALTHY EATING

The foods people eat can affect mood. People may crave unhealthy, high-fat foods when stressed. But eating these foods can worsen mental health. They can make people feel tired. People may skip meals because of stress. Hunger also has a negative impact on mood.

A healthy diet can reduce anxiety. People should eat foods that are rich in nutrients. Protein gives people energy. Complex carbohydrates also provide an energy boost. Oatmeal and whole grains are rich in these nutrients. People should avoid foods that have a lot of sugar.

It is also important that people drink water. Not having enough water can affect mood. People should limit caffeine intake. High levels of caffeine can worsen symptoms of anxiety. They can also make it difficult to fall asleep.

MEDITATION

Some people meditate to cope with stress and anxiety. Meditation allows people

VITAMINS

Some studies have shown that low levels of vitamin D lead to anxiety. Vitamin D helps with mood. Sunlight helps the body produce vitamin D. Foods such as salmon are another source of this vitamin. Some cereals and orange juices are also enhanced with vitamin D.

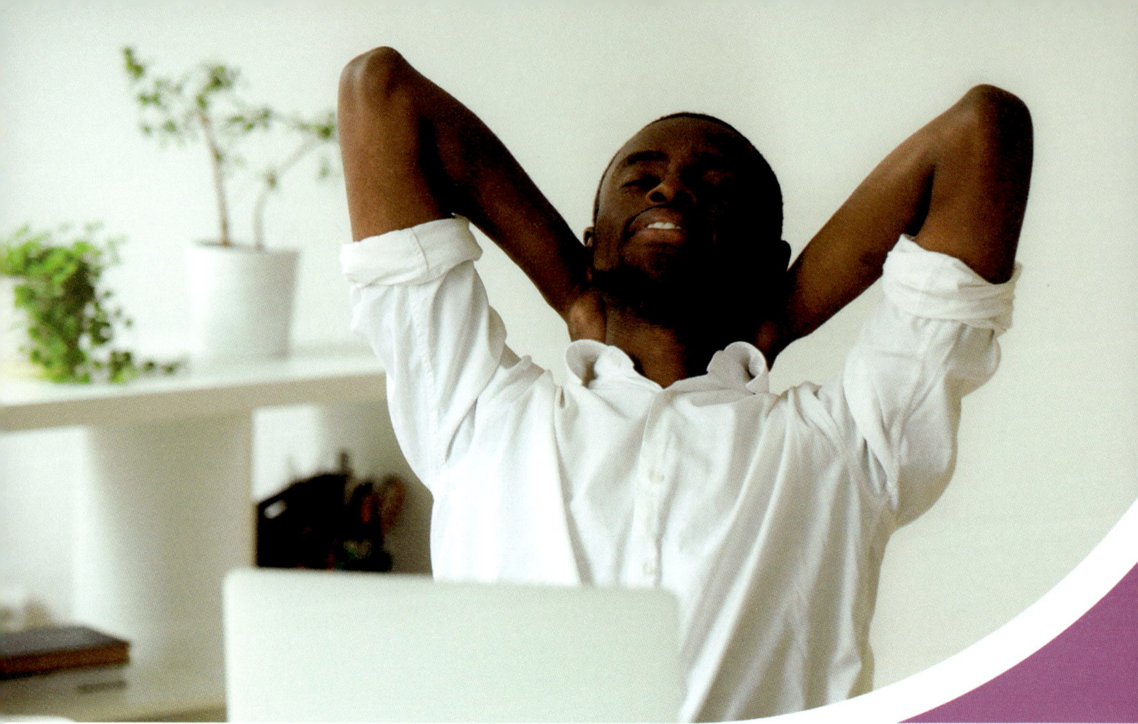

to practice clearing their minds. They

may form a different relationship with

their anxiety.

Some people pay attention to what their

bodies are feeling. They think about the

space around them. This can help prevent

them from being overwhelmed by anxiety.

Deep-breathing exercises have a similar effect. People take shallow breaths when they are panicked. Mindful breathing helps people take deep, even breaths. This can reduce feelings of anxiety. Even five minutes of meditation can lower stress levels.

Treating an anxiety disorder takes patience and commitment. But medication and therapies are effective treatments. People with anxiety disorders can boost these treatments with lifestyle changes. With proper treatment and management, people with anxiety disorders can have happy, full lives.

GLOSSARY

addictive

having qualities that make it difficult to stop the use of a drug or a behavior

diagnosis

an official identification of a disorder or disease made by a doctor

dose

how much of a medication is taken and how often it is taken

hormone

a chemical produced by the body that can affect mood or behavior

neurotransmitter

a chemical substance that is produced in the brain and nerves

prescribe

to officially recommend a medication or treatment

symptoms

signs of a disease or disorder

withdrawal

the symptoms and feelings caused by stopping the use of an addictive drug

SOURCE NOTES

INTRODUCTION: A NEW SCHOOL

1. Quoted in Psych Hub, "How Do I Help My Child Cope with Anxiety?" *YouTube*, December 22, 2020. www.youtube.com.

CHAPTER ONE: HOW DOES ANXIETY FEEL?

2. Quoted in Michelle Crouch, "This Is What a Panic Attack Feels Like," *AARP*, May 2, 2022. www.aarp.org.

CHAPTER TWO: THERAPIES TO TREAT ANXIETY

3. Quoted in "CBT for Anxiety: How It Works & Examples," *Choosing Therapy*, January 5, 2023. www.choosingtherapy.com.

4. Quoted in Emily Laurence, "How to Overcome Social Anxiety, According to Experts," *Forbes*, October 19, 2022. www.forbes.com.

CHAPTER THREE: TREATING ANXIETY WITH MEDICATION

5. Quoted in International OCD Foundation, "How Long Should a Child Take Medication for Anxiety/OCD?" *YouTube*, November 12, 2018. www.youtube.com.

CHAPTER FOUR: LIFESTYLE CHANGES TO REDUCE ANXIETY

6. Quoted in Lindsey Konkel, "Which Medications Are Best for Anxiety Disorders?" *Everyday Health*, April 8, 2021. www.everydayhealth.com.

BOOKS

Katie Kawa, *What Happens When Someone Has Anxiety?* New York: KidHaven Publishing, 2020.

Cherry Pedrick and Bruce M. Hyman, *More Than Stress: Understanding Anxiety Disorders*. Minneapolis, MN: Twenty-First Century Books, 2023.

Maddie Spalding, *Understanding Phobias*. San Diego, CA: BrightPoint Press, 2022.

INTERNET SOURCES

"Anxiety," *TeensHealth*, March 2022. https://kidshealth.org.

"Anxiety Disorders," *Mayo Clinic*, 2022. www.mayoclinic.org.

"Cognitive Behavioral Therapy," *Psychology Today*, 2022. www.psychologytoday.com.

Anxiety in the Classroom – I Am a Student
https://anxietyintheclassroom.org/student

Anxiety in the Classroom offers resources to students about how to manage and talk about anxiety in school. It also shares information about how friends and siblings can support loved ones who have an anxiety disorder.

Mental Health America
https://mhanational.org

Mental Health America is an organization that is dedicated to the prevention, diagnosis, and treatment of mental health disorders. Its website includes information about mental health and tools to promote a mentally healthy life.

National Alliance on Mental Illness
https://nami.org

The National Alliance on Mental Illness raises awareness about mental health. Its website provides resources to help people understand symptoms of mental health disorders, including anxiety disorders. It aims to support and educate people with mental illnesses.

INDEX

Sheryl Normandeau is a writer based in Calgary, Alberta, Canada. Her nonfiction and fiction work has been published internationally.